MR. SPECIAL HELPS
MRS. PRECIOUS COMPLETE
A TOTAL TRANSFORMATION

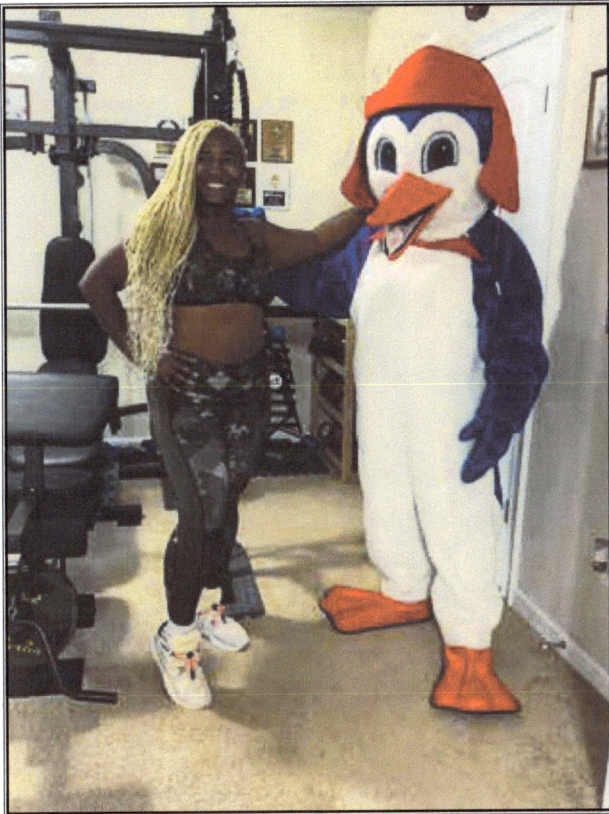

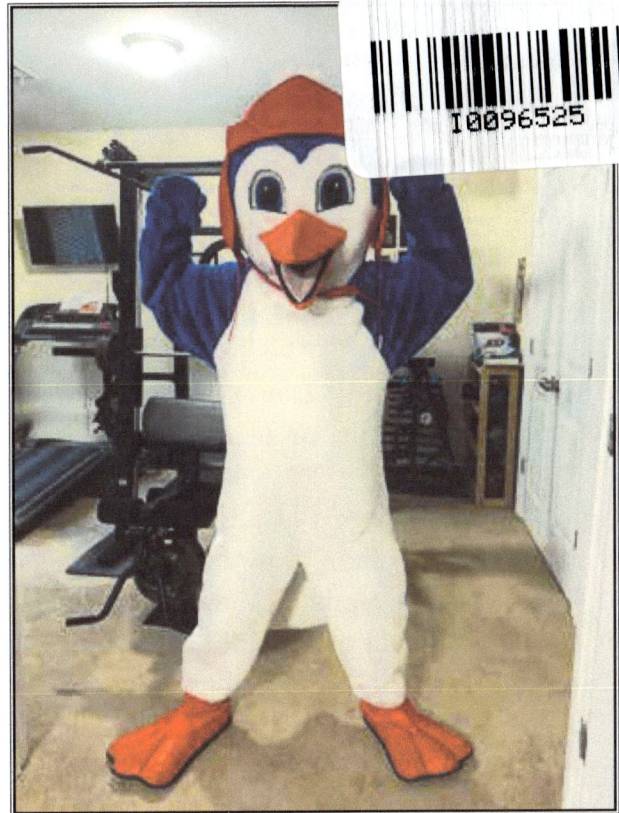

SHARON JENISE HALL

Mr. Special Helps Mrs. Precious Complete a Total Transformation
Copyright © 2022 by Sharon Jenise Hall

ISBN
978-1-958690-20-8 (Paperback)
978-1-958690-21-5 (eBook)

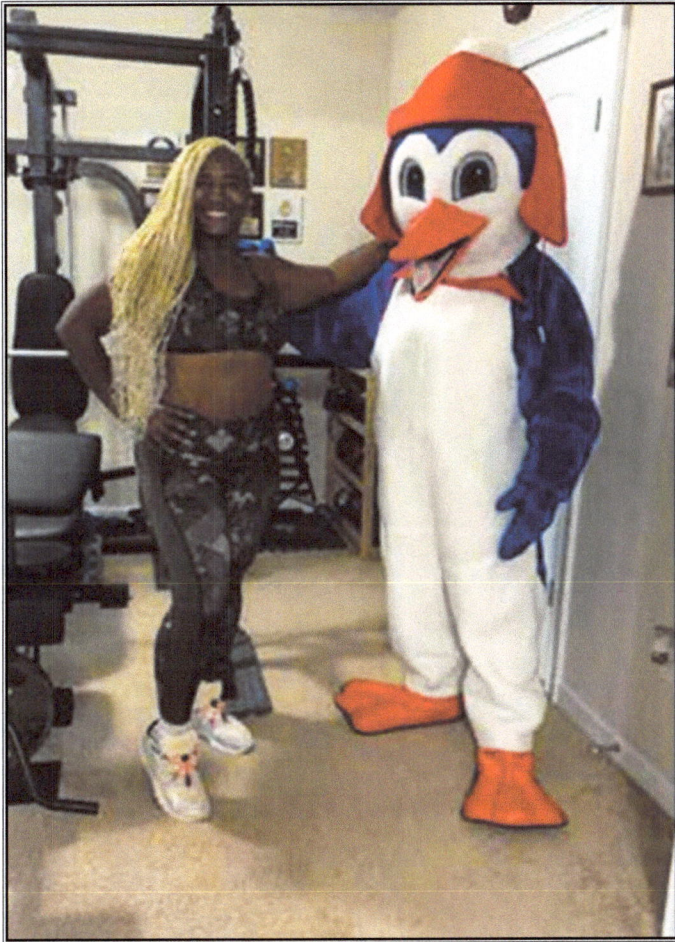
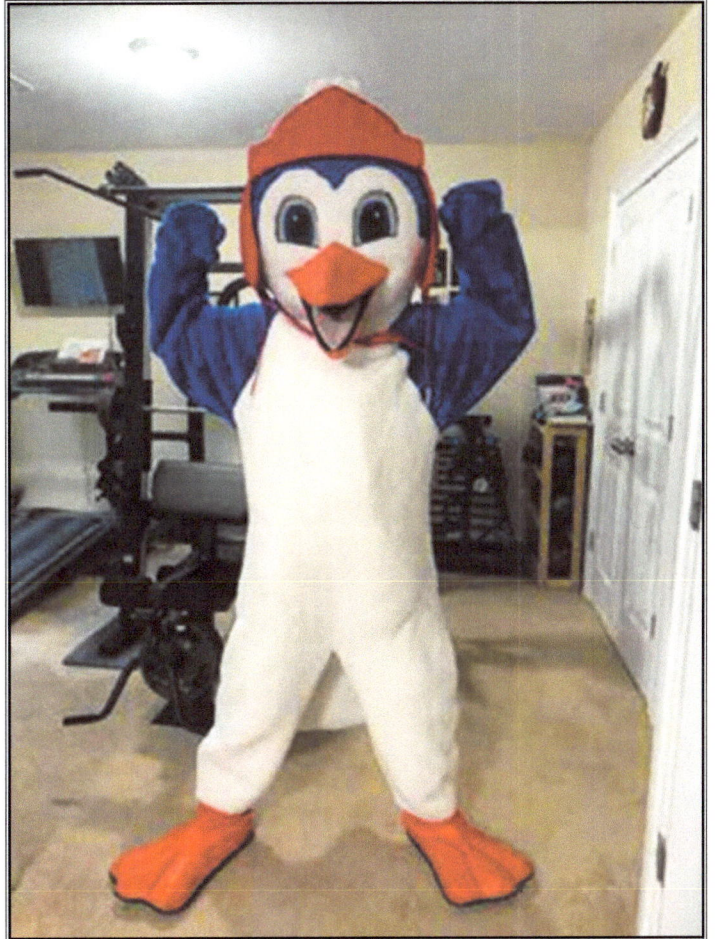

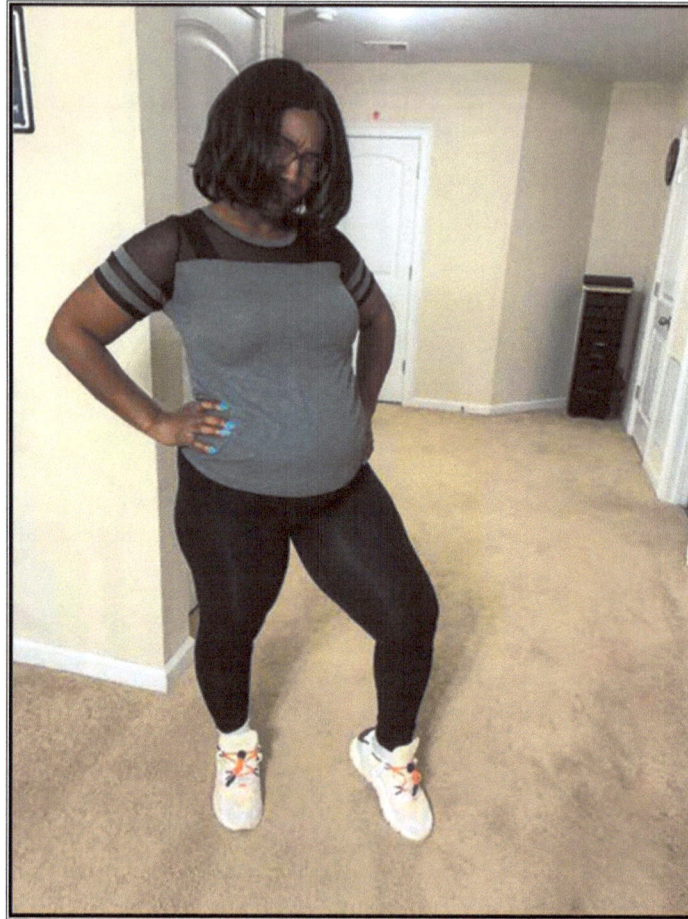

After several months into the pandemic, Mrs. Precious felt a certain way.

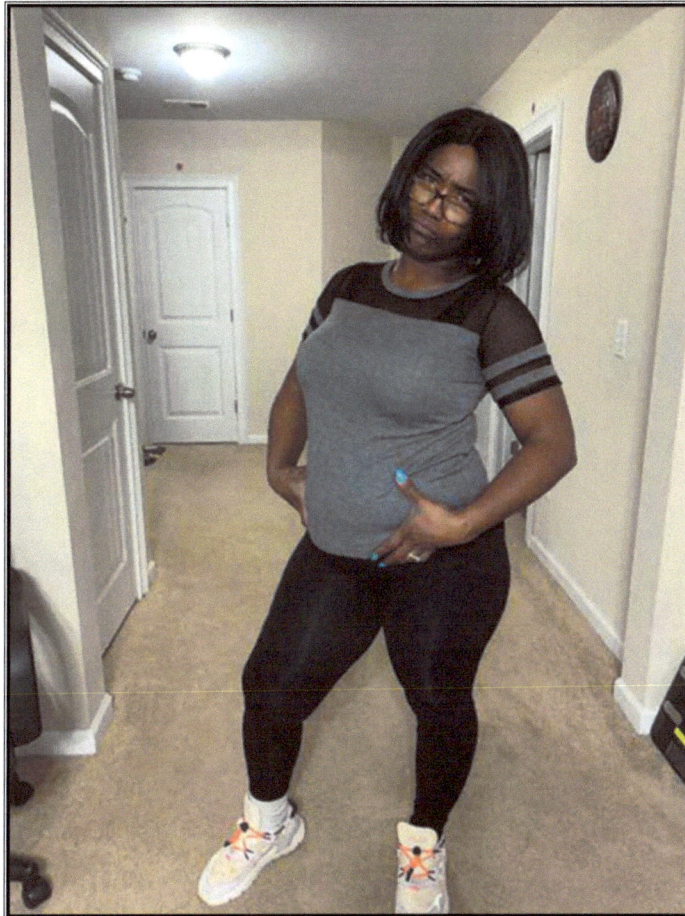

She wanted to change everything about herself, including her mind, body, and soul. Mrs. Precious wanted to change every aspect of her being.

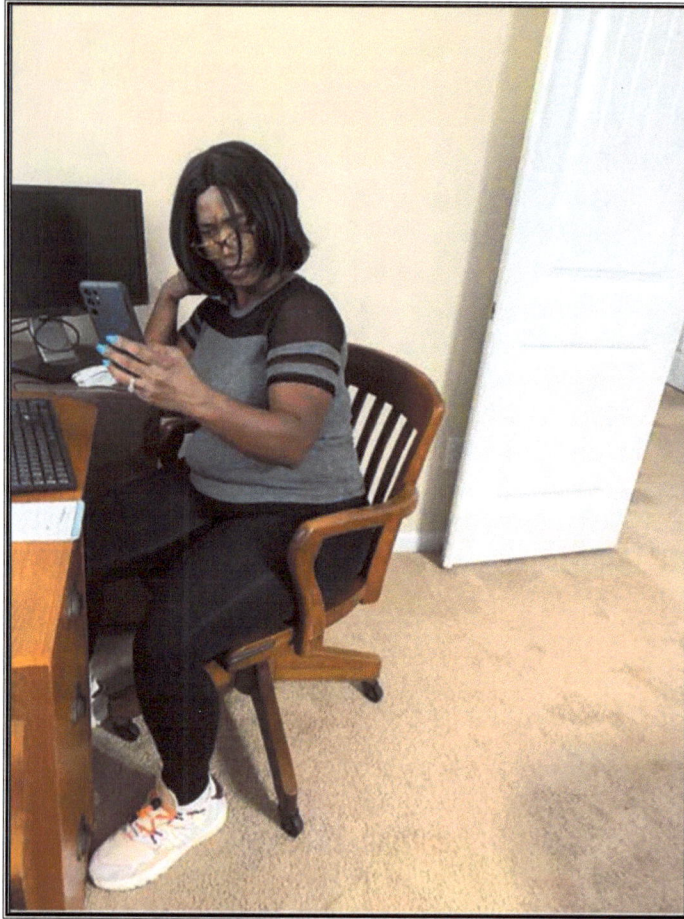

Mrs. Precious thought, Let me call on Mr. Special for help. She did just that.

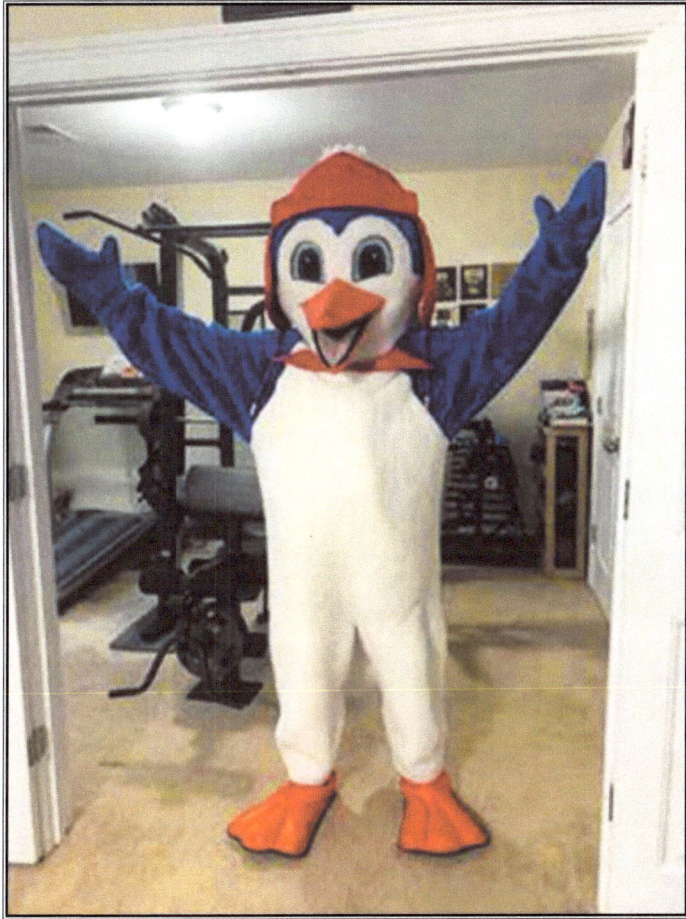

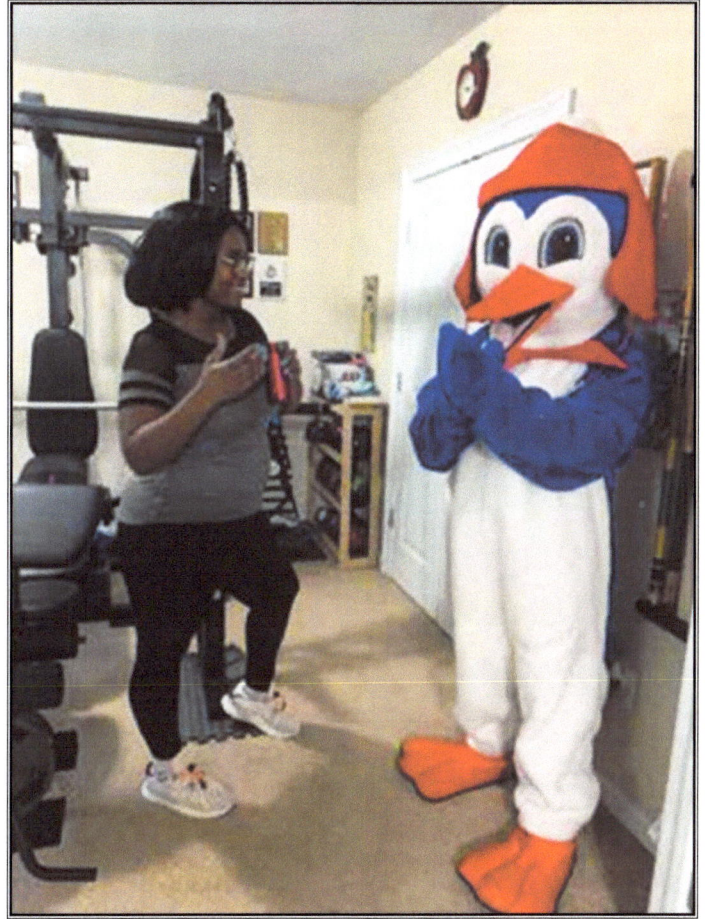

Mr. Special felt moved with compassion to assist Mrs. Precious quickly.

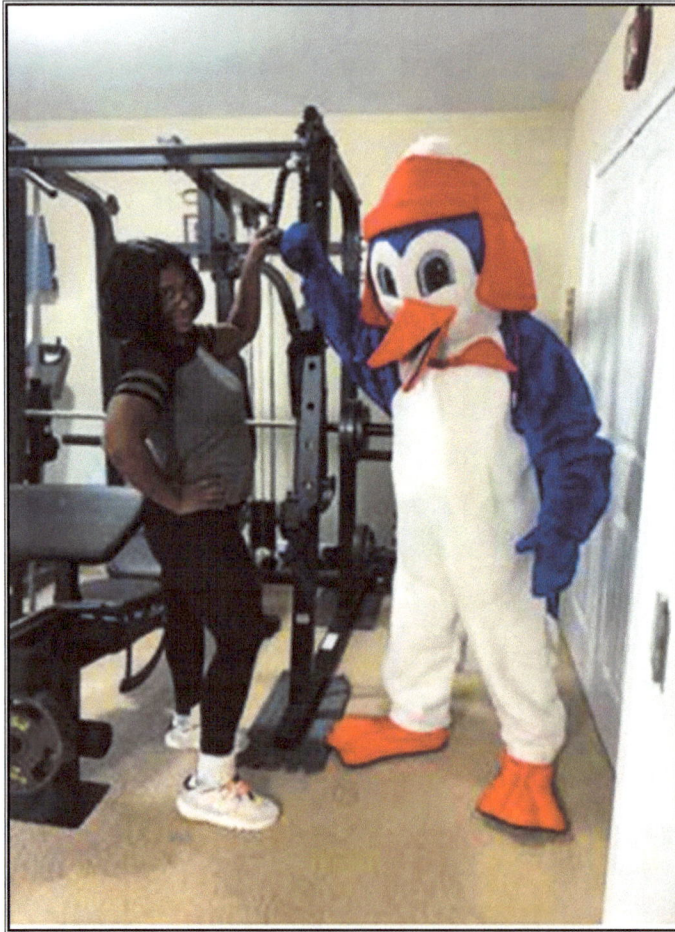

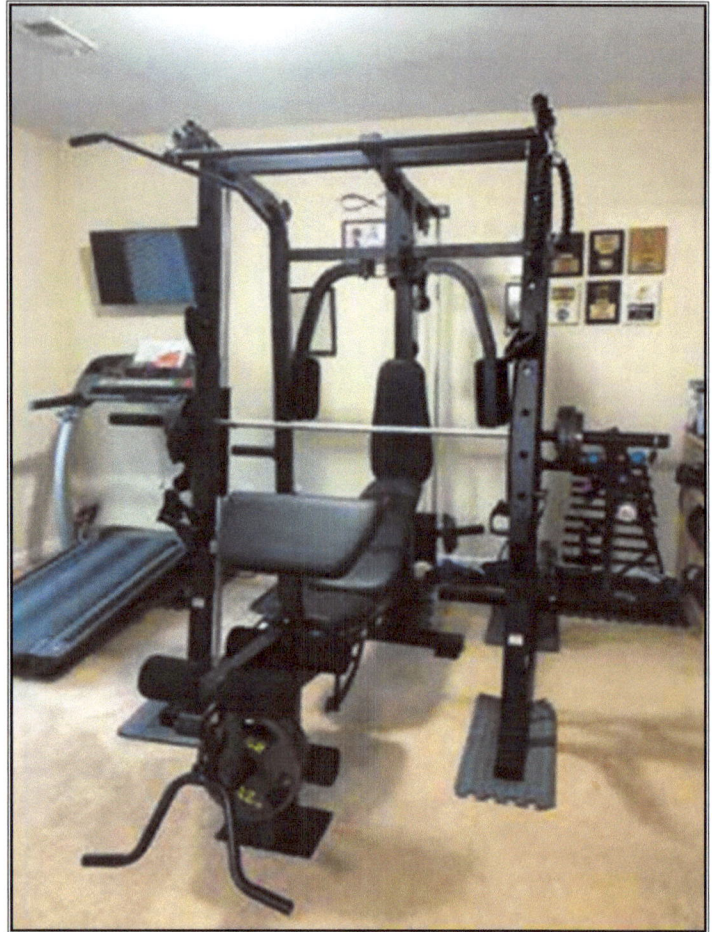

Mrs. Precious wanted to start by changing her physical appearance first. Mr. Special suggested to start out by working out at the gym.

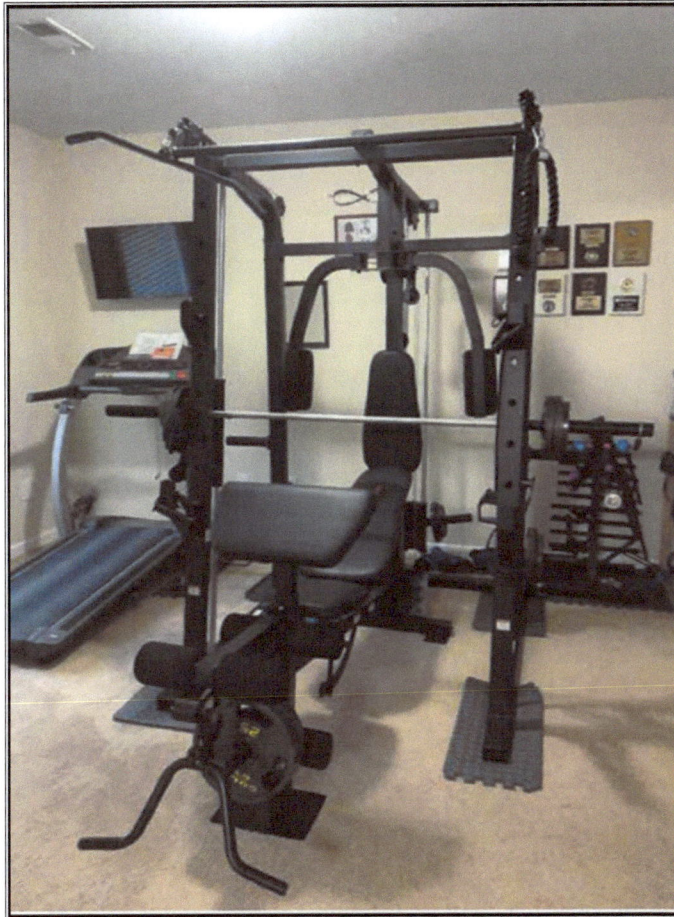

A few times a week will be a good start.

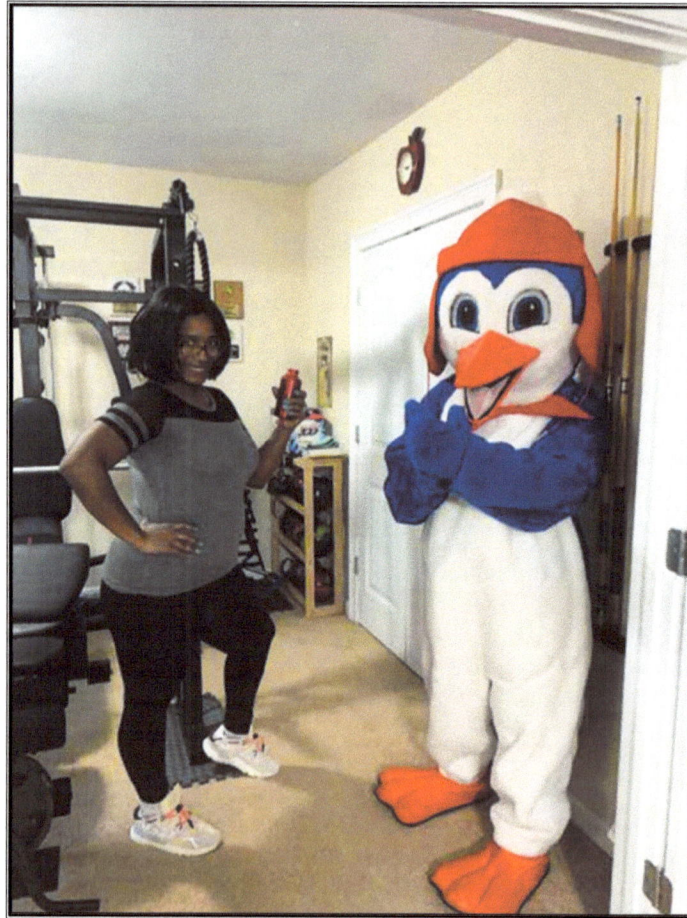

Mr. Special created a well-balanced diet to go along with the exercise program for six weeks and a workout schedule for Mrs. Precious for six months.

MEAL PLAN

Monday			
Breakfast	Lunch	Dinner	Morning/ Evening Snack
1-2 waffles	1 cup green salad	1 cup green salad 4	1 apple 1/4 cup almonds 1 cup skim milk
8 oz. glass orange juice	1/2 cup green peppers 1 whole grain roll cabbage, celery, carrots, 1 cup green beans	oz. codfish 1 medium potato	

Tuesday			
Breakfast	Lunch	Dinner	Morning/ Evening Snack
1 cup rice 2 small pancakes 1 cup skim milk	1/4 cup cottage cheese 1 cup peaches 1 cup green salad	1 cup green salad 1 cup green beans 3 oz. sirloin steak	6 oz. fat-free yogurt 1 orange

Wednesday			
Breakfast	Lunch	Dinner	Morning/ Evening Snack
1 bagel 1 T light cream cheese 1 cup orange juice	2 oz. turkey breast 1 large whole grain 2 carrots slice, 1 cup skim milk Thursday	1 cup angel pasta 2 oz. boiled shrimp 1 tsp. olive oil w/ garlic on pasta	1 cup fat-free pudding 1 apple 1 mixed green salad, 1 cup green beans

Thursday			
Breakfast	Lunch	Dinner	Morning/ Evening Snack
1 French toast 1 cup strawberries 1 cup skim milk	2 oz. lean hamburger 1/2 slice tomato 1/4 slice green pepper	2 slices cheese pizza 1 large mixed green salad 1 T fat-free dressing	1 orange 6 oz. fat-free yogurt 1 T ketchup

Friday

Breakfast	Lunch	Dinner	Morning/Evening Snack
1/2 cup cooked oatmeal 2 tsp. brown sugar	2 oz. turkey breast 1/2 cup skim milk 1/2 cup orange juice	1 oz. chicken breast, no skin milkshake 1 apple 1 small baked potato Saturday	1 low fat 1 pear 1 cup mixed green salad

Saturday

Breakfast	Lunch	Dinner	Morning/Evening Snack
1/2 English muffin 1 egg poached 1/2 grapefruit 1 cup skim milk	1 cup mixed green salad 1 T fat-free dressing 3 oz. albacore tuna 6 crackers	1 cup pasta 1/2 cup spaghetti sauce 1 mixed green salad 1 T fat-free dressing, 1 cup skim milk	1/2 oz. chocolate 1 whole graham cracker 1 apple

Sunday			
Breakfast	Lunch	Dinner	Morning/ Evening Snack
1 cup cereal 1 cup skim milk 1 cup blueberries 1/2 cup orange juice	1 cup vegetable soup 1 cup mixed green salad 1 T fat-free dressing 6 crackers	1 piece flounder 1 cup rice 1 cup mixed green salad	1 apple 3 cups light popcorn 1 cup carrot

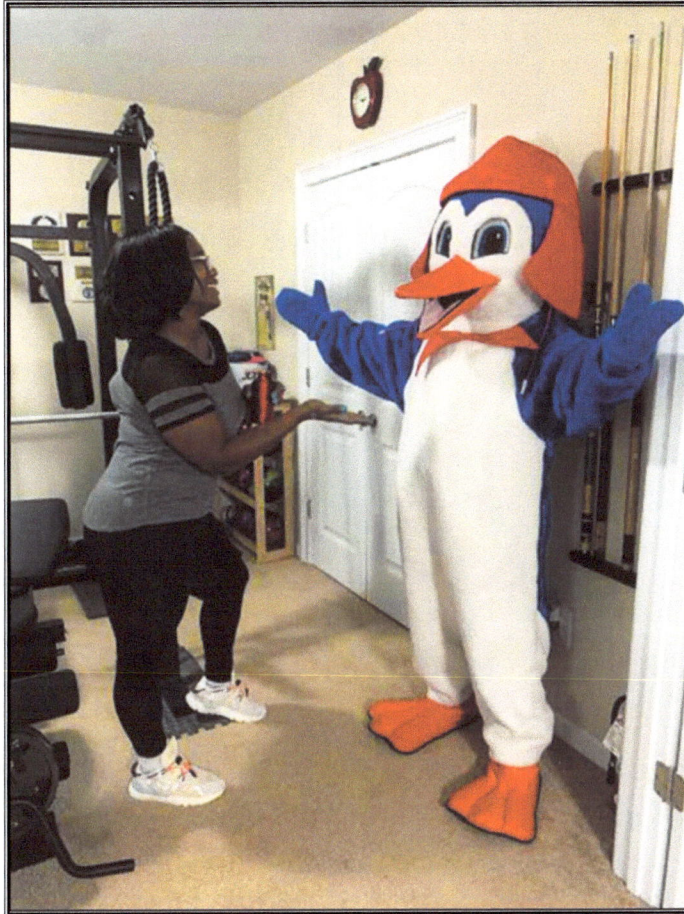

Mrs. Precious agreed upon the total transformation
with the help of Mr. Special.

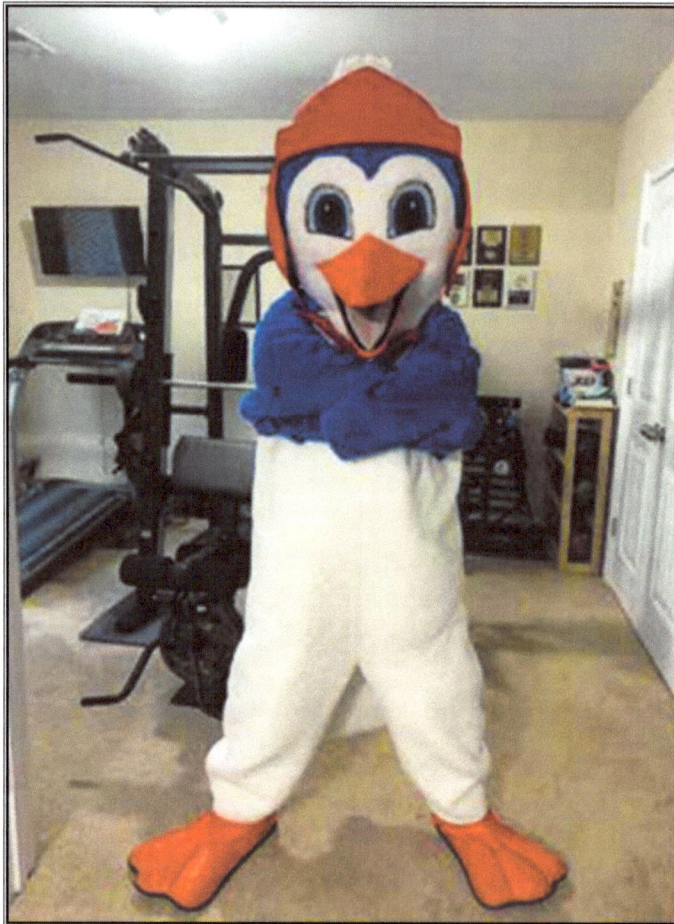
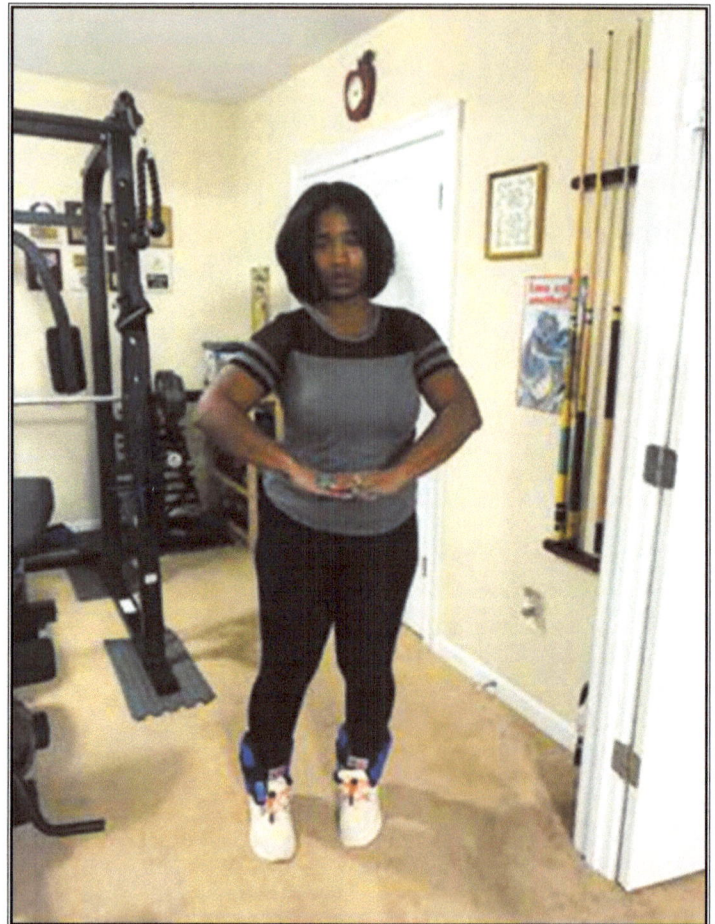

Mr. Special met Mrs. Precious on Monday at the gym, and the total transformation started!

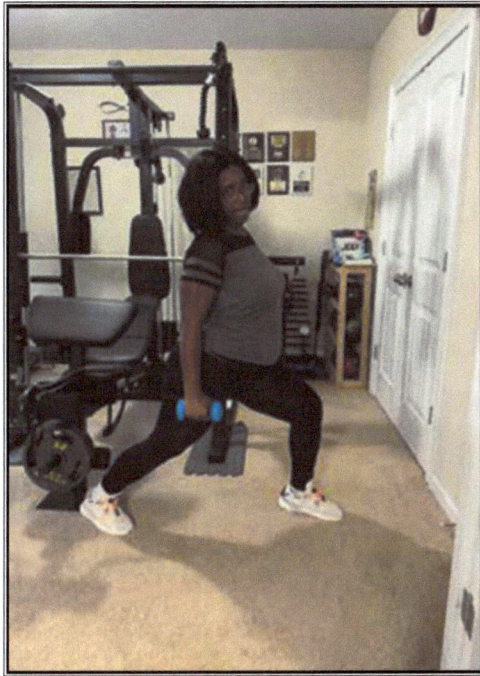

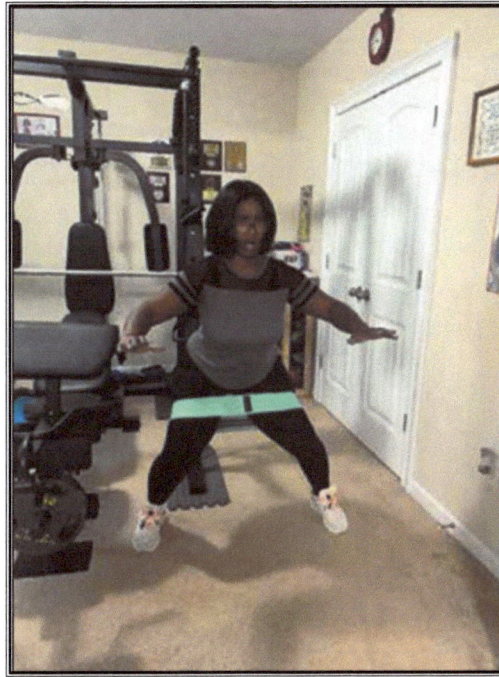

Exercises for Legs	
Lying Lateral	Goblet Squat
Leg Raise	Banded Lateral Walk
Isometric Squat	Single-Leg Dead Lift
Stability Ball	Sumo Dead Lift
Mini Band Clamshells	Stability Ball Bridge
Mini Band Kickback	Lateral Lunge with Balance
Banded Glute Bridge	Squat with Heel Raise
Bulgarian Split Squat	Suitcase Dead Lift
Stability Ball Hip Thrust	Sumo Squat
Reverse Lunge	Isometric Calf Raise
Duck Walks	Supported Single-Leg Dead Lift
Step-up	Curtsy Lunge
Lateral Step-out Squat	Pistol Squat

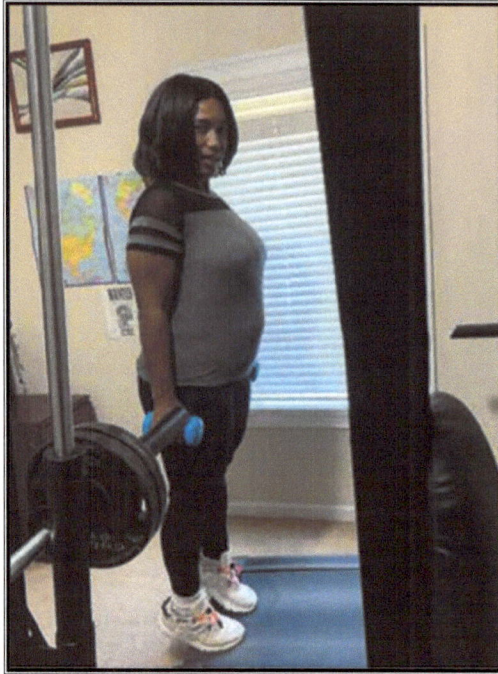

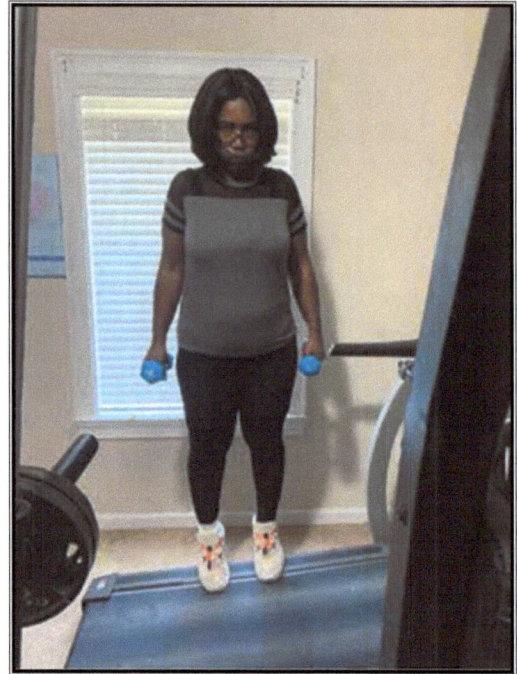

Other Exercise Movements	
Mountain Climbers—20 seconds	High Knees—20 seconds
Crab Toe Touches—20 seconds	Jump Lunges—20 seconds
Repeat	Repeat
Push-up Side Plank—20 seconds	
Plank Hip Rolls—20 seconds	
Repeat	
Note: 30 seconds' rest between each set	

On Wednesday, Mrs. Precious and Mr. Special worked on arms and other movement.

Exercises for Arms	
Hammer Curls	Wide Grip Curl
Chin-up	Pullover/Triceps Extension
Suspension Trainer	Standing Dumbbell Fly
Neutral Grip Triceps Extension	Decline Triceps Extension
Inverted Row	Lying Triceps Extension
Close Grip Push-up	High Pull
Behind the Back-Cable Curl	Overhead Press
Close Grip Curl	Conventional Curl
Dip	Side Curl with Band
Diamond Push-up	Close-Grip Bench Press
Pound Stone Curl	Face Pull
Suspension Trainer Biceps Curl	Tate Press
Reverse Curl	Band Lateral Raise

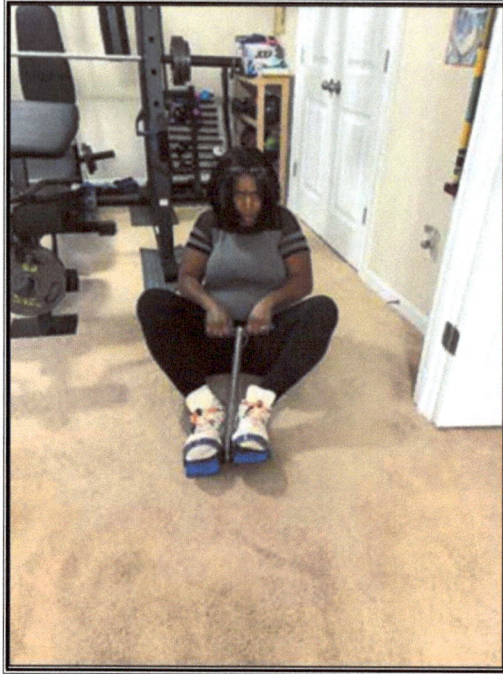
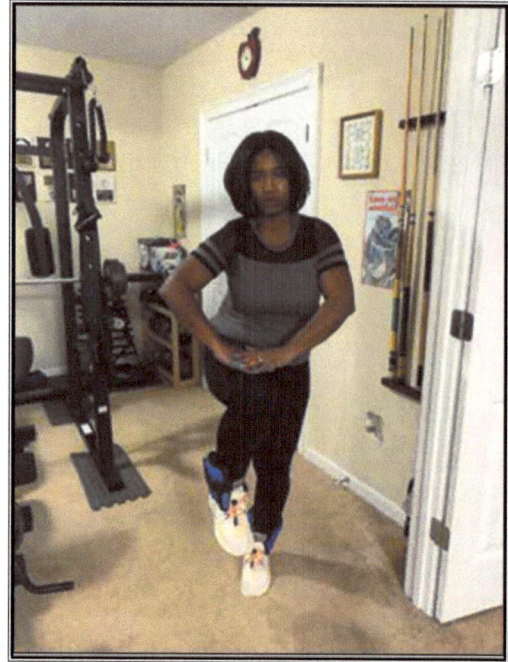

Other Exercise Movement

Straight Leg Calf Raise—4 sets of 15 reps
Kettlebell Hip Thrusts—4 sets of 15 reps
Barbell Rolls—4 sets of 15 reps
Leg Press—4 sets of 15 reps
Single-Leg Split Squats—4 set of 15 reps
Note: 2-3 minutes' rest between each set

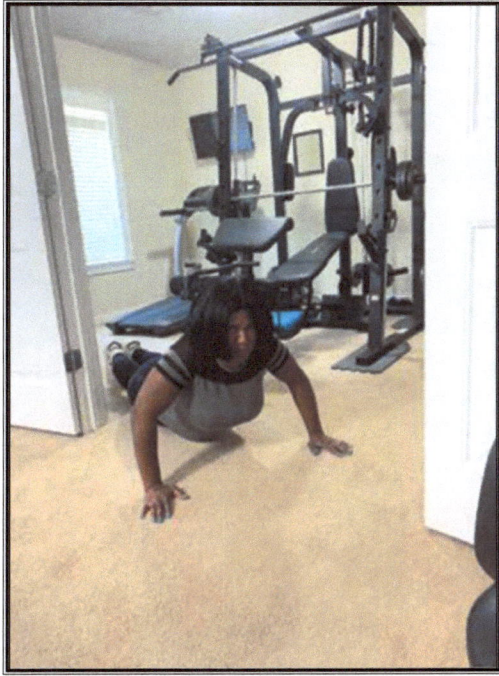

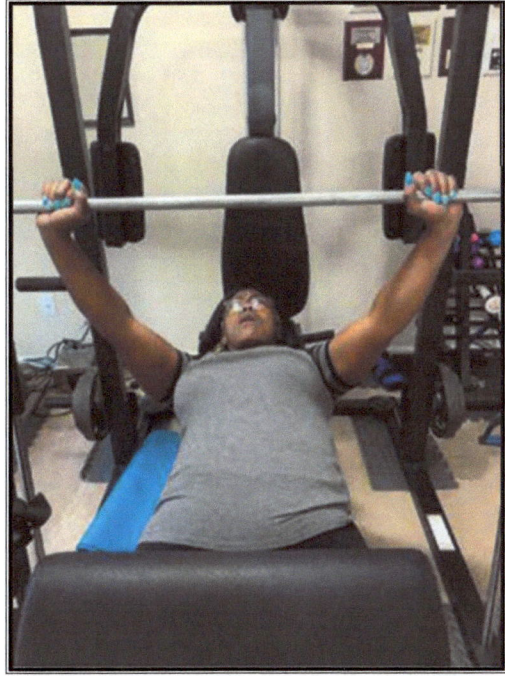

On Friday, Mr. Special and Mrs. Precious worked on total body and other movements.

Exercises for Full Body	
Push up	Step-ups
Squats	Pull-ups
Burpees	Dips
Lunges	Jump Lunges
Running and Cycling	Stair Climbing
Mountain Climbing	Leg Raises
Kettlebell Swings	Handstand
Box Jumps	

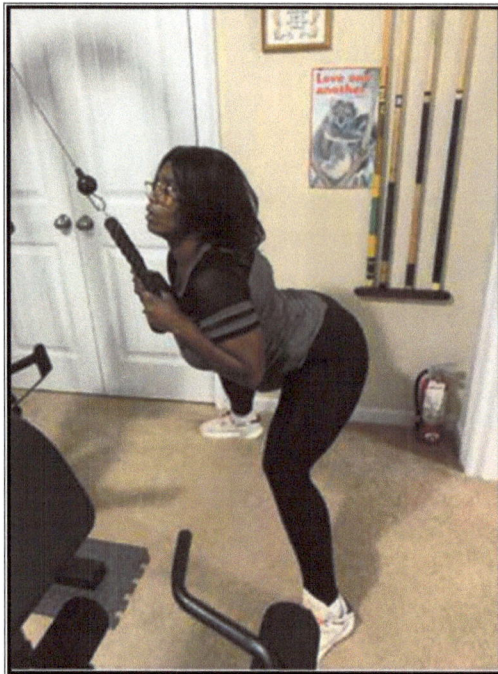

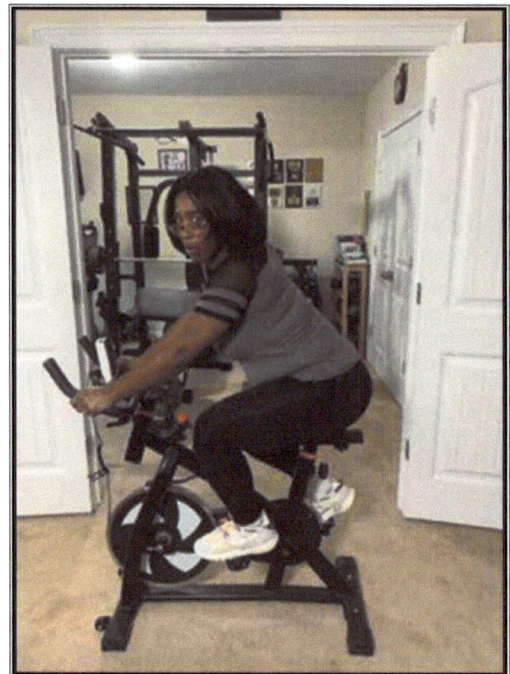

Other Exercise Movement	
Mountain Climbers—20 seconds Crab Toe Touches—20 seconds Repeat Push-up Side Plank—20 seconds Plank Hip Rolls—20 seconds Repeat Note: 30 seconds' rest between each set	High Knees—20 seconds Jump Lunges—20 seconds Repeat

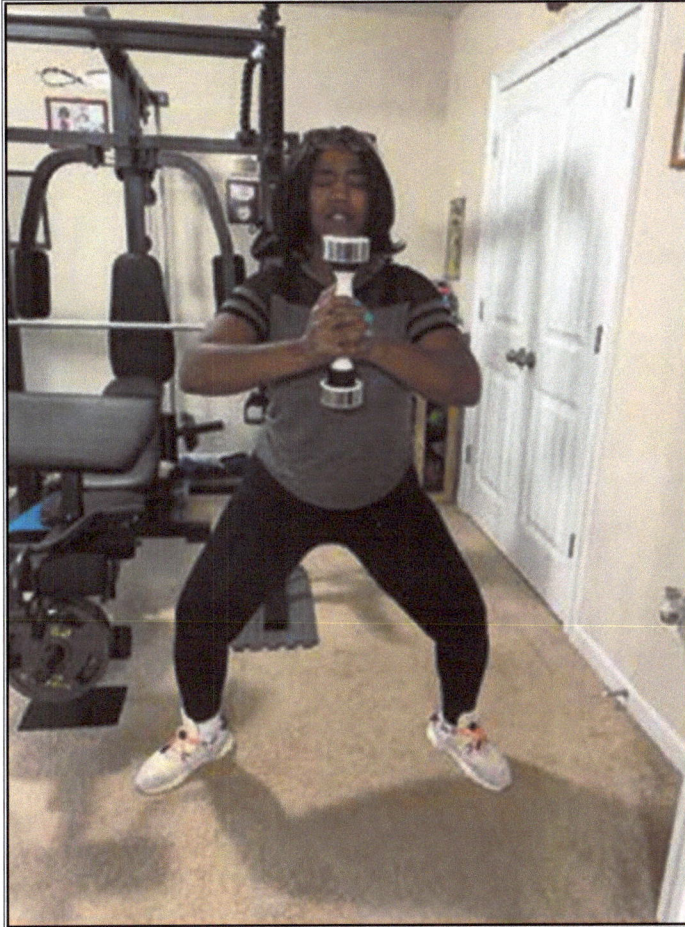
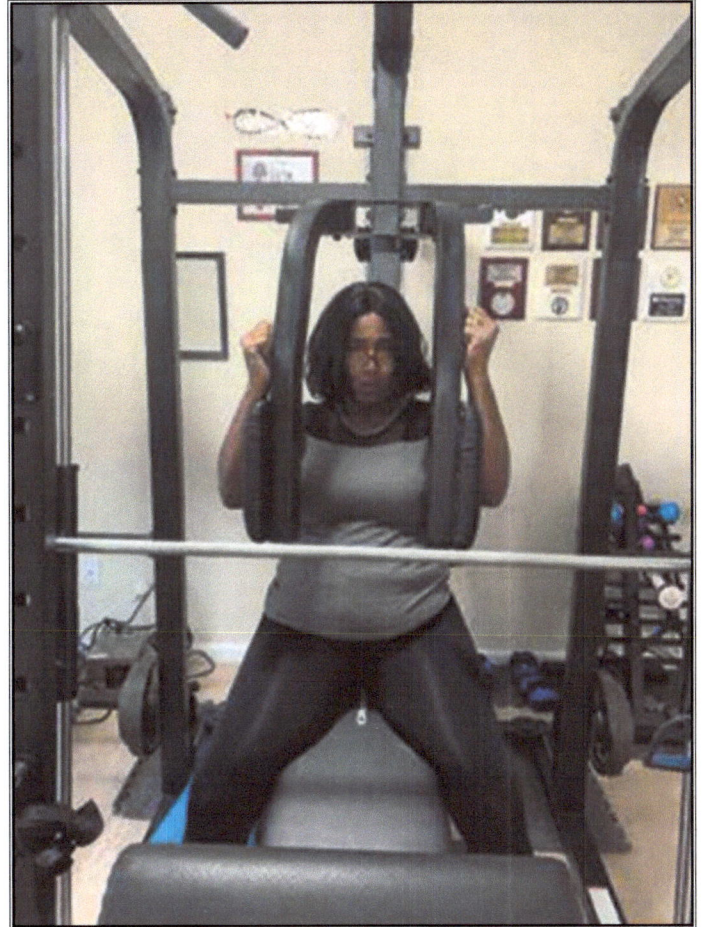

These routines continued for six months.

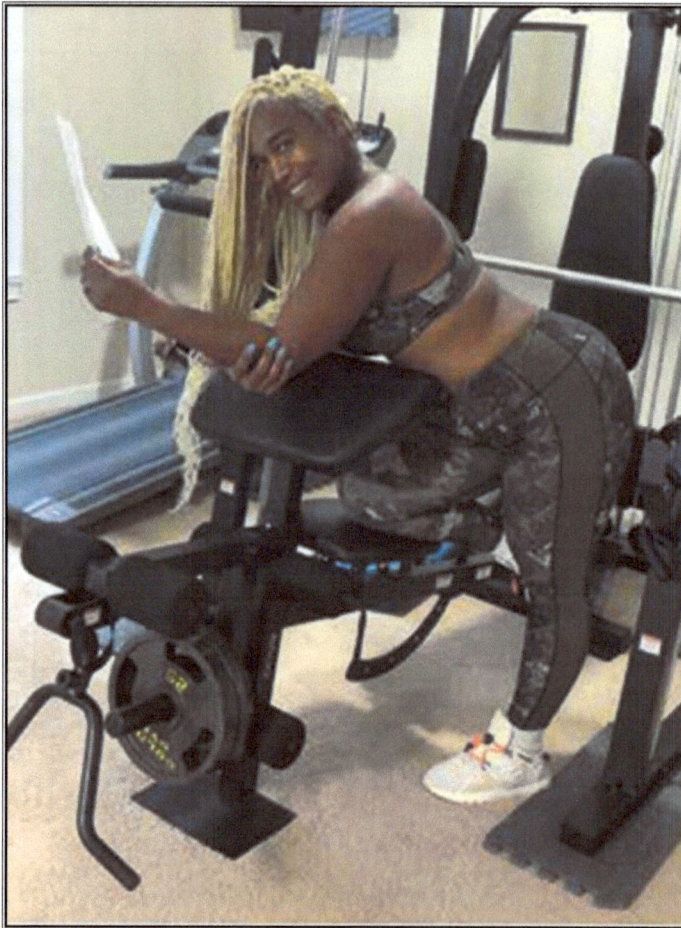

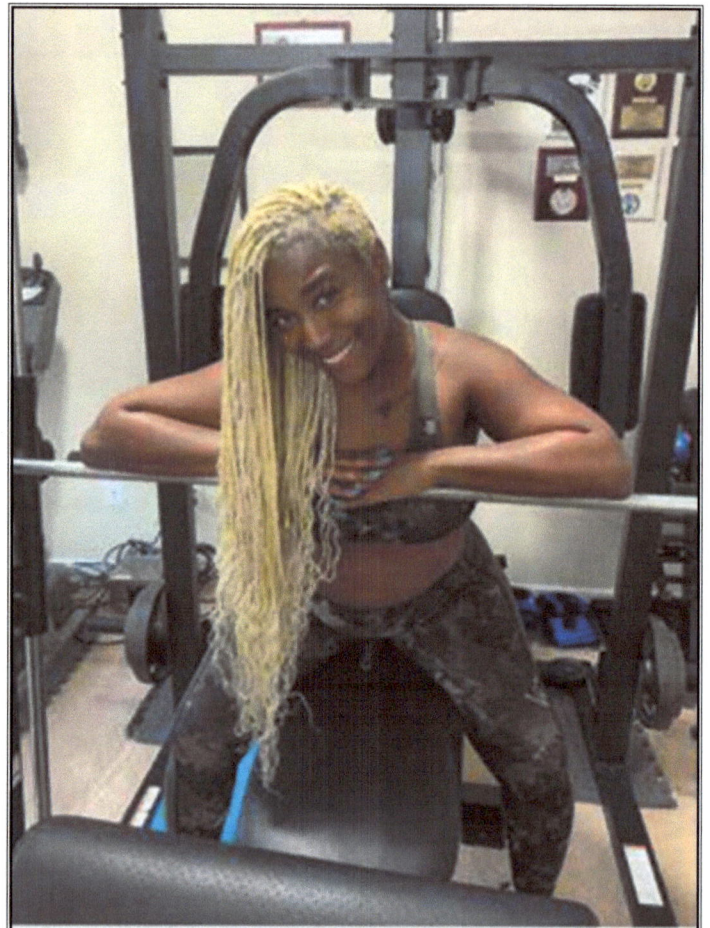

Now, Mrs. Precious was very happy with the results of the transformation of her body.

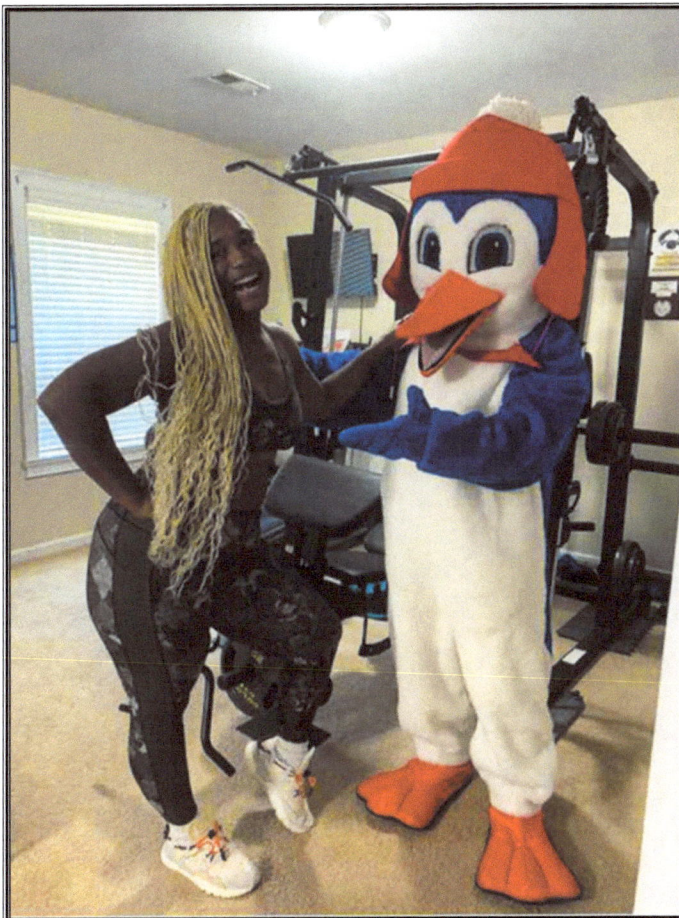

She was so happy that she wanted to transform her facial looks and hair color.

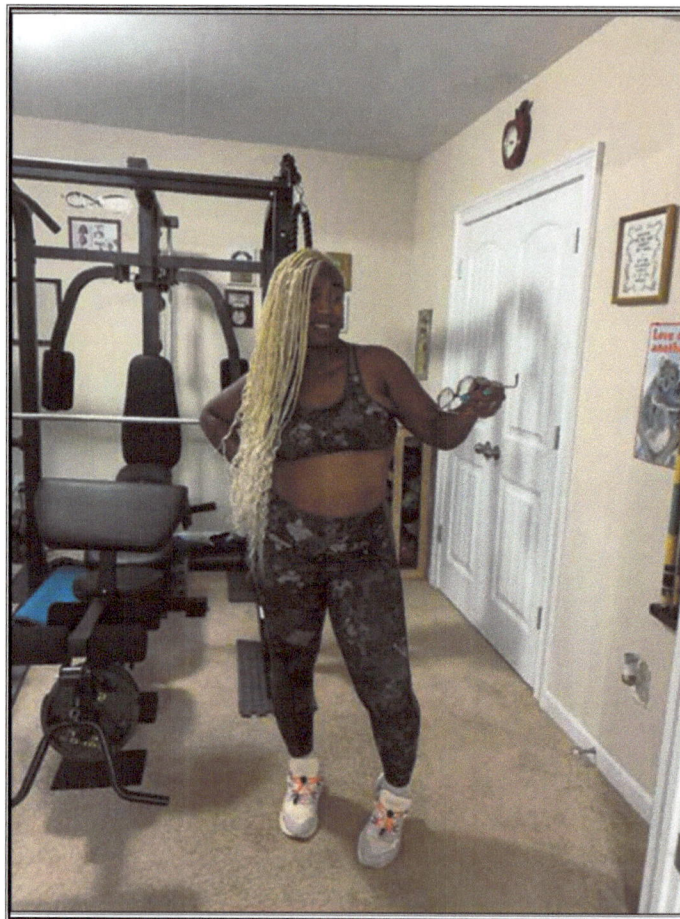

She said, "Away with the glasses," and she started wearing contacts.

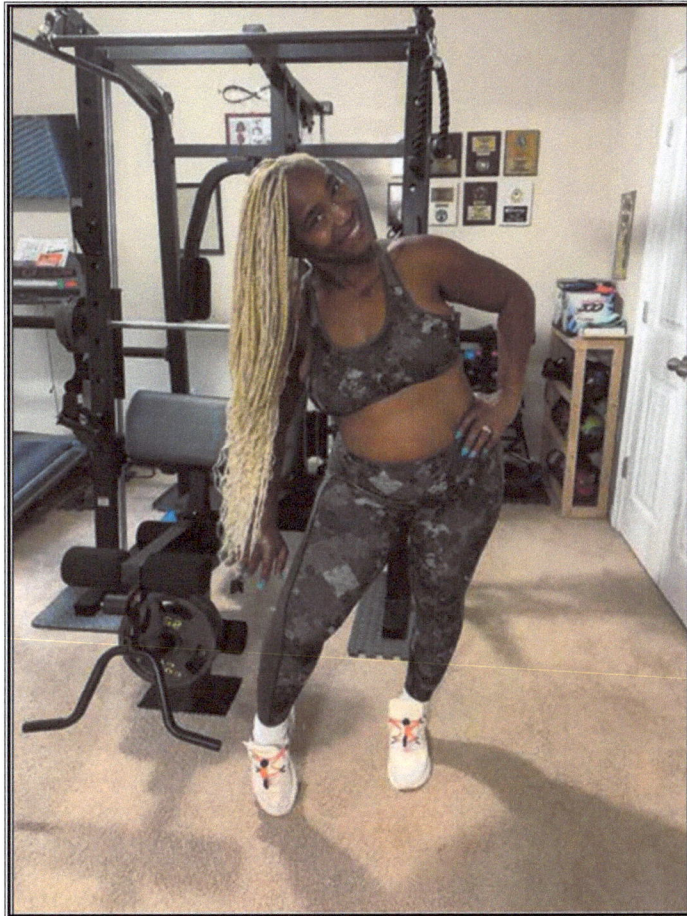

She said, "Let me bring some light to my hair and make my hair bright."

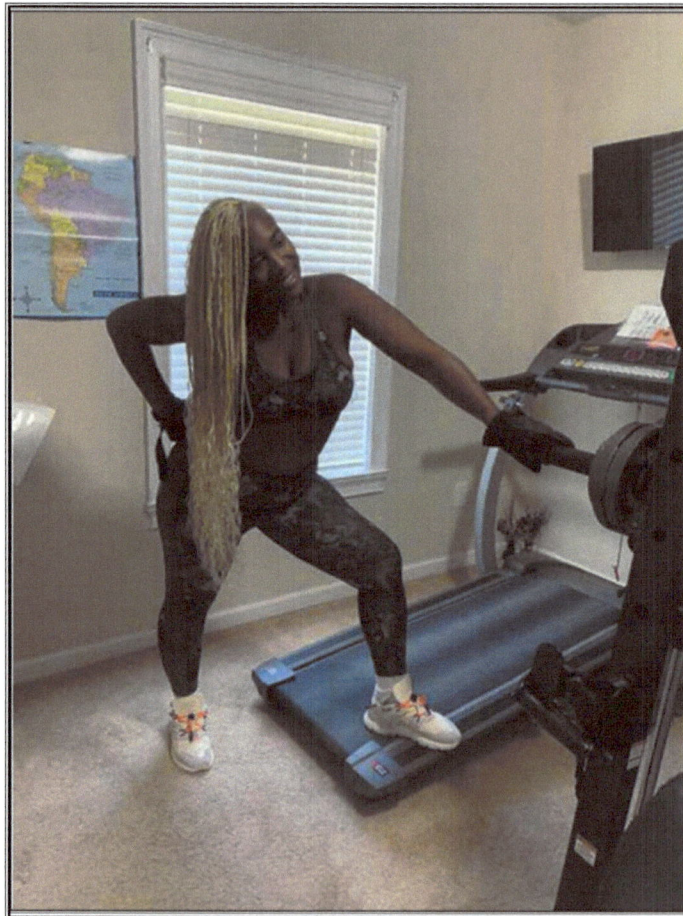

Mrs. Precious was really starting to like the total transformation of her body.

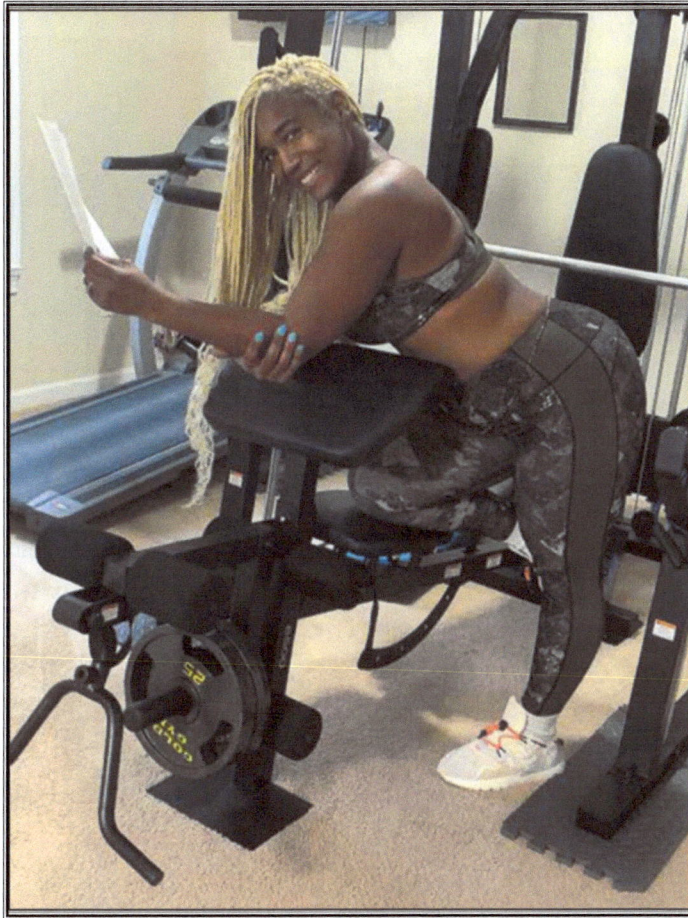

After the six months of exercising and eating a well-balanced diet, taking off the glasses and coloring her hair, Mrs. Precious was very happy with the total transformation of her body.

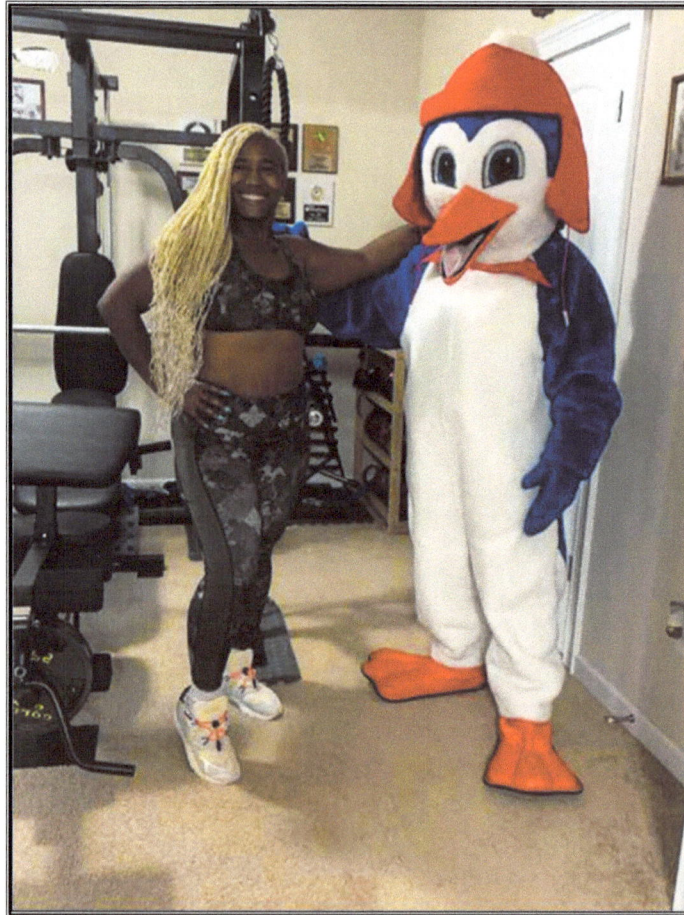

After the six months of exercising and eating a well-balanced diet, taking off the glasses and coloring her hair, Mrs. Precious was very happy with the total transformation of her body.

www.ingramcontent.com/pod-product-compliance
Lightning Source LLC
Chambersburg PA
CBHW061147030426
42335CB00002B/130